IS YOUR GARDEN A DA

If you are new to the idea of c
facts to consider.

MW01612406

HERBICIDES DON'T JUST KILL WEEDS

Commonly used herbicides have actually been shown to be toxic to both animals and plants. The startling results of one study showed that dogs that play in herbicide-treated yards have a 300% increased risk of cancer. Another study links herbicides with non-Hodgkin's lymphoma cancer in humans. A manufacturer-supported review of studies found a widely-used herbicide safe for use around humans, although certain studies found that it can affect human embryonic, placental, and umbilical cells *in vitro*.[2]

PESTICIDES DON'T JUST KILL GARDEN PESTS

Pesticides sprayed or sprinkled in your garden do not discriminate; they are lethal to all things that crawl, slither, squirm, or fly in or around your garden. However, only about 1% of insects that come around your garden are actually a concern to the average gardener. Treating with pesticides disrupts the natural ecosystem of the garden by exterminating both pollinators and beneficial insects along with the destructive ones. What's worse is that once you eradicate all insects from your garden, you basically open it up for even more damaging pests to invade, often resulting in a population explosion that is worse than the original problem. Pesticides are like antibiotics in this way; they serve to create stronger, genetically advanced, pesticide-resistant pests.[2]

As if that weren't enough, pesticides harm our environment as they contaminate soil, groundwater, surface streams, and the air. Many common pesticides have been shown to contain dangerous neurotoxins, as well as hormone-disrupting agents and even carcinogens. Recent studies have shown pesticides can be held at least partially responsible for a myriad of health concerns, including asthma, fertility issues, neurological disorders, Parkinson's disease, bronchitis, neuroblastoma, leukemia, and autism.[2]

WHAT'S REALLY IN YOUR FERTILIZER?

Every good gardener knows fertilizing a garden is important to provide proper nutrition to plants, flowers, shrubs, and trees. However, synthetic, chemical-based fertilizers are not as beneficial as one may think. Inorganic fertilizers are often made from industrial waste and can contain dangerous substances such as nitrates, lead, arsenic, cadmium, and even some radioactive components.[3] These things are not only damaging to plants, but they contaminate the soil and groundwater supply. When these contaminated waters run off into ponds, lakes, and streams, they upset delicate ecosystems by over-stimulating algae growth, which in turn suffocates other aquatic plants, invertebrates, and fish.[2]

The Environmental Protection Agency (or EPA) conducts ongoing research on the safety of many common garden pesticides, herbicides, and fertilizers. The EPA website lists dozens of chemicals that are undergoing review for their short-term effects on people, animals, and the environment. While it is known that many of these chemicals are hazardous in large doses, little is known about the long-term consequences of using the products according to recommended dosages on product labels. Individual chemicals that are deemed safe by the EPA may still be a danger when combined.[3] Studies are showing that an ever-growing number of chemicals are considered hormone disruptors. Hormone disruptors can throw off the body's natural hormone balance, often leading to certain types of cancer.[2]

These are just some of the reasons why many people are resorting to organic methods for their gardens. Why take a chance by spraying your fruits and vegetables with harmful carcinogenic chemicals? Why risk contaminating your water supply or destroying a local ecosystem? Organic gardening is a responsible alternative that produces healthy, vibrant results.

Growing organically is more than just avoiding the use of synthetic fertilizers and pesticides; it involves creating a healthy environment where plants thrive, and where pests and weeds are controlled with natural substances that maintain balance and do not disrupt the natural ecosystem of the environment.

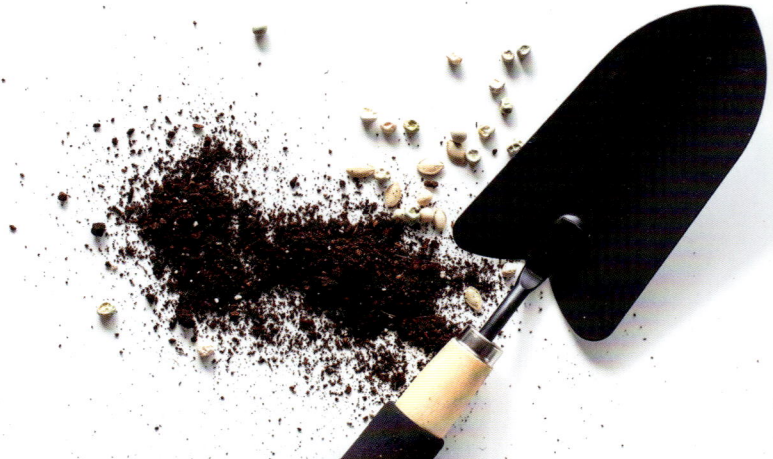

Essential Oils in the Garden

WHAT ARE ESSENTIAL OILS?

Essential oils are the life force of plants. These concentrated, natural, and aromatic liquids are extracted from shrubs, flowers, trees, roots, and leaves. Plants depend on their essential oil to grow and adapt to their surroundings. Within the plant, essential oils play a very important role by protecting against pests, disease, and harsh environmental conditions. Every drop of essential oil has a very complex chemical make-up containing hundreds of active constituents that work together in harmony to create the immune system of the plant.

Because they are natural and easily recognized by our cells, people have been using essential oils for centuries as a means of alternative medicine and aromatherapy. It just makes sense that we can use these very same substances to protect and heal the plants from which they are obtained.

Essential oils can be valuable gardening tools for anyone interested in organic gardening. They are very effective at chasing away harmful garden pests, protecting plants against disease, improving the health and growth of plants, and attracting beneficial insects. The gardener reaps many rewards from a healthy garden treated with natural essential oils.

In the pages of this book, you will learn how to eliminate nasty, chemical fertilizers, insecticides, and other toxic chemicals from your garden and replace them with pure, natural essential oil recipes and remedies. There is even a section that will give you tips and tricks for using essential oils to clean garden tools and the greenhouse, as well as a few recipes designed to pamper the gardener after a satisfying day working in the garden. From prepping your garden plot to harvesting your bounty, the recipes and methods in this book will help you get on the path to a cleaner, safer, more satisfying gardening experience.

FIRST THINGS FIRST — SAFETY TIPS

- Do not apply essential oils to plants when the temperature is over 100°F. To prevent doing this, the ideal time to apply essential oils is in the morning.
- Do not apply essential oils to plants if plant tissues are wet or if rain is likely.
- Avoid spraying plants with essential oils in the fall before winter hardening has occurred.
- Do not apply essential oils to plants along with sulfur or sulfur-containing pesticides.
- Certain plants tend to be sensitive to essential oils. In these cases, it is best to avoid direct application. Oils may be diluted and sprayed on the soil around plants to avoid over-treating. A few examples are: Black Walnut, Douglas Fir, hickories, junipers & cedars, maples (especially Japanese and Red Maples), Red Bud, Smoke Tree, spruce (esp. Dwarf Alberta Spruce).
- Do not spray essential oils while pets are nearby as they can be sensitive to certain oils.
- If essential oil gets in the eye, flush with a mild carrier oil such as olive, coconut, or almond oil. Rinsing with water will only serve to increase discomfort.
- Store your oils in a cool, dark place. Light, air exposure, and heat can cause oxidation and destruction of some active constituents in essential oils.

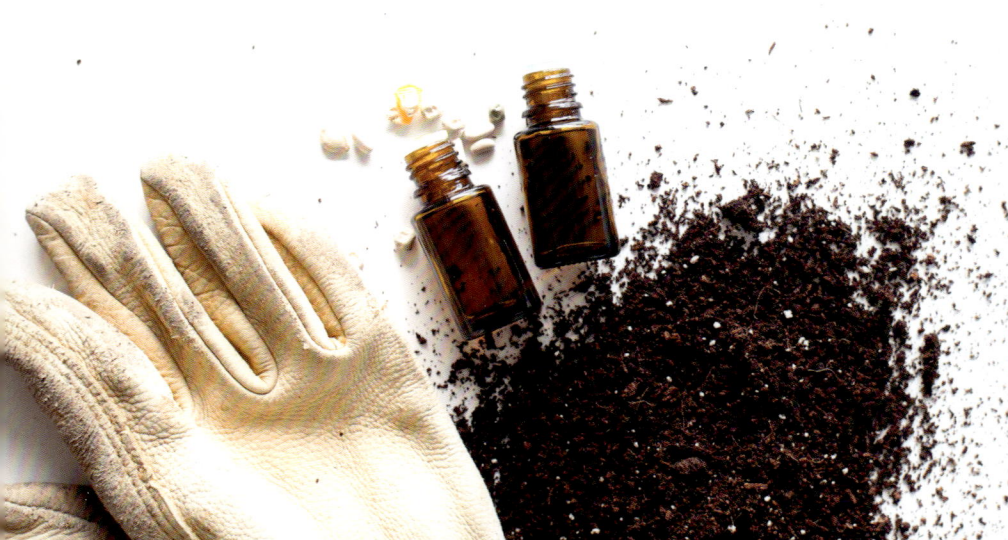

Organic Gardening Tips for Beginners

We all want the food we serve our families to be as healthy as possible. Organic gardening provides a means of growing healthy, high quality foods and flowers without the use of synthetic chemicals. Organic methods are healthier, better for the environment and wildlife, and less expensive because there are no chemical fertilizers, pesticides or herbicides to buy. All of this is accomplished by working with nature instead of against it. While many think starting their own organic garden is complicated, the truth is anyone with a little time, a small growing area, and a passion for good food can grow a garden. All you need is patience and willingness to weed and water. You can get started by following a few basic guidelines:[4]

1. PICK YOUR PLOT

- **Size:** Think small, especially at first. A small garden takes less work and fewer materials.

- **Location:** Most warm-season vegetables need at least six-hours of full sun each day. However, even if you don't have an area in full sun, you can still grow some vegetables. Most gardeners prefer their potted vegetables or raised bed gardens close to their house for more convenient harvesting when cooking. Choose a spot that is close to a water spigot for frequent watering.

- **Method:** The most popular choices for garden plots are directly in the ground, in raised beds, and container gardening.

  - **The ground** is often the most economic location, since you don't have to purchase containers or soil. Growing straight in the ground also offers the benefits of resident organisms that will help your garden thrive.

  - **Raised beds** are the way to go if your existing soil quality is poor, and you want to start planting right away. The beds can be bordered with materials such as brick, untreated wood, or stone to separate it from potential contaminants. You will want to keep the beds narrow so you can reach the middle; four-feet is a good width, and sixteen-inches is an ideal height. Simply build your frame, fill the bed with soil and compost, and you are ready to plant.

- **Container gardening** is a great option for growing many plants in a small space. Tomatoes, green onions, peppers, beans, and lettuce do particularly well in containers. Use large containers as they provide greater reserves of nutrients and water and allow space for roots to grow. Make sure containers have holes in the base to allow for adequate drainage.

2. PREPARE THE SOIL

Healthy plants need healthy soil. Soil is the most important aspect when it comes to organic gardening.

- **Humus**
  Organic soil is rich in humus—the result of decaying materials such as leaves, grass clippings, and compost. It helps to retain moisture and allows for sufficient drainage.

- **Beneficial organisms**
  Organic soil is alive and will support living organisms such as earthworms, nematodes, fungi, protozoa and bacteria, all of which help maintain the quality of the soil.

- **Nutrients & pH**
  Your soil should be loose and airy and have plenty of essential minerals. Proper pH is a vital characteristic of healthy soil. Most minerals and nutrients are best available to plants in soils with a pH between 6.5-6.8. There are 17 or so elements thought to be essential for plant growth. Nitrogen, phosphorus, and potassium are the most vital, while calcium, magnesium, and sulfur are known as secondary nutrients also important to many plants.

  One way to determine the mineral content of your soil is to have it tested. Basic do-it-yourself kits are available at most gardening and home improvement stores, or you can obtain a more thorough, low-cost test from your local county cooperative extension office or university. You can find the extension service for any location here: https://www.gardeningknowhow.com/extension-search/

- **Compost:** Compost combines fertilizer, mulch, and weed preventer in an all-in-one mixture. If you don't have a compost pile, you can purchase compost by the bag or truckload. To improve your soil, spread a two- to four-inch layer of compost, decayed leaves, dry grass clippings, or manure over the entire surface of your garden.

When using manure in your garden, be sure it has aged at least a year and that it is exclusively from plant-eating animals like cows, sheep, goats, and chickens. Never use fresh manure or that from carnivorous animals. Compost is the organic gardener's best friend, and an annual application of compost will improve most any soil.

- **Fertilizer:** Good fertilizer adds essential nutrients that might not be readily available in your soil. Organic garden fertilizers slowly release nutrients into the soil. Avoid harsh, synthetic fertilizers that are harmful to the environment and can kill off beneficial microorganisms.

3. PLANT SELECTION

No matter how great your soil is, if you don't choose the right plants for your area, they won't thrive. After testing your soil, carefully choose plants that will be well suited to each location based on the moisture, drainage, amount of sunlight, and soil quality. The healthier your plants are, the more resistant they will be to disease and pests. It's important to check the USDA's Hardiness Zone Map (found at http://planthardiness. ars.usda.gov/PHZMWeb/) to find which plants will grow well in your area. Be sure to seek out only certified organic plants, seedlings, and/or seeds. The best variety and selection of plants suited for your area can often be found at your local garden center or farmer's market.

4. PROPER PLANTING

After you have chosen your plants, follow instructions on the labels regarding spacing and planting methods specific to each type of plant. Make sure there is ample space between plants to promote air circulation

Making your own compost can be easy!

You need carbon-rich materials such as garden trimmings, dry leaves, straw, wood chips, and sawdust. These are the "brown" sources. Nitrogen-rich materials, such as grass clippings, green leaves, plant material, livestock manure, coffee grounds, and kitchen waste, are the "green" sources. Do not use animal products or dairy in your compost pile as they may rot and attract scavengers. Choose a suitable location or bin for your compost pile. Layer brown and green materials at a 3-to-1 ratio with a little soil between each layer. Keep the pile moist and turn it at least every week or two. In a few months, you should have dark, crumbly compost that smells like fresh earth.[5]

and avoid fungal attacks. Grouping your plants will help to reduce weeding, wasting of water, and will make it easier to apply compost.

5. PROPER WATERING

Whether you water by hand or install an irrigation system, the best time to water is in the morning. Mornings tend to be cool and less windy, so less water is lost to evaporation. Avoid watering at night as this can lead to fungal and bacterial diseases. Apply water near the base of plants for absorption by the roots. Avoid spraying the leaves, which can be easily damaged. It is better to deep-water your plants a couple of times a week than to shallow-water every day. Most experts recommend a total of about one-inch of water per week (including rainfall). To conserve water and help plants, consider collecting rainwater to use in your garden.

6. WEEDING

Weeds siphon water and nutrients from your garden, harbor pests, and detract from the beauty of your garden. Combining a natural approach with the following tips will help keep your garden weed-free. Hand-weeding is the preferred method to remove weeds because it eliminates the use of chemicals, and it gives you the opportunity to get some exercise while working in the garden. Compost will help cut down on weeds, as will organic mulch, which also helps protect the soil. Over time, mulch will decompose into the soil and provide additional nutrition.

7. PROTECT PLANTS FROM PESTS

Bugs are a part of a gardener's everyday life. Encourage beneficial insects and pest predators such as toads, frogs, lizards, birds, bats, spiders, and ladybugs to hang out in your garden. This will help control pests and diseases without the use of chemical pesticides. A safe method to deal with limited infestations is to simply remove larger insects and caterpillars by hand. Companion planting involves selecting and growing a variety of companion crops that support the growth of your garden while keeping pests and weeds away. Maintaining a clean garden will prevent many pests from invading your garden. Even with proper precautions, the occasional infestation is to be expected. There are many natural pesticides that can be made using essential oils and other ingredients from your kitchen. (See the Organic Pest Control section on p. 12.)

8. HARVESTING

Finally, all the work has paid off, and you get to reap the benefits of your labor! Harvesting provides the most rewarding experience after you have spent so much time and energy nurturing your garden. A crop requires consistent harvesting to continue producing. With many crops, the more you harvest, the more your plants will produce for you.

After distillation, Young Living recycles plant material by adding it to compost piles along with animal manure, leaves, grass, and any clippings from the farms. They also have worm houses at many farms, where they not only reproduce beneficial earthworms, but also have a system for collecting worm castings. Even the liquid byproduct from this process is utilized as a nutrient-rich spray for plants at the farms.[6,7]

Organic gardening is full of rewards, providing healthy food for your family while caring for the health of the environment as well. By following these easy steps, you can be well on your way to harvesting your first meal straight out of your very own garden. The more you care for your garden, the better it will bloom and produce for you.

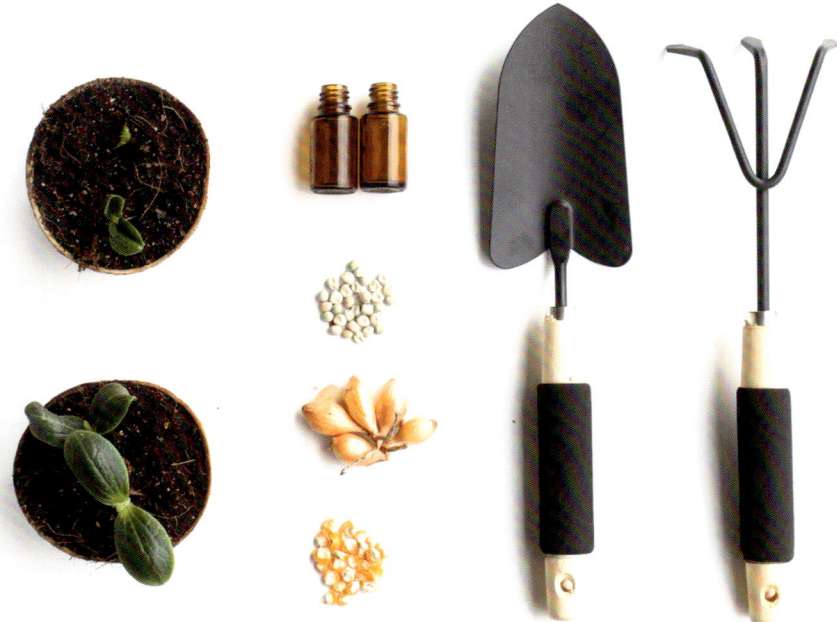

Organic Pest Control with Essential Oils

Essential oils are very effective at keeping the garden pest and chemical free. Based on the pest you are trying to control or eliminate, choose one or more essential oils from the list below and apply according to one of the following application methods:

ESSENTIAL OIL SPRAY:
- Best to deter insects.
- Add 8-10 drops of desired essential oil to a gallon of water and spray directly on plants or the soil around them. This is the best method to use as a deterrent, treating for disease, and to encourage plant growth.

COTTON BALLS:
- Best to deter ground-moving insects, mice, squirrels, cats, and dogs.
- Add 4-5 drops of essential oil to cotton balls and scatter around the area or place in burrows or nests. You can also place the cotton balls in small containers and bury the container in the ground, keeping the top level with the soil.

HANGING STRIPS OF CLOTH:
- Best to dissuade cats, dogs, and other animals from entering the garden. This method can also be used to attract pollinators and beneficial insects.
- Spray a solution of water and essential oils on cloth strips and hang from stakes, dowels, or other structures.

STRING:
- Best to deter flying insects.
- Soak a string in a solution of water and essential oils, and string between rows of plants.

COMMON GARDEN PESTS:

Ants—While ants do not cause harm to plants, they do encourage aphids by protecting the aphids from beneficial predators. Fire ants can pose a hazard simply because of their painful bite.[8]

Look for: anthills on the ground; small holes in the ground with displaced dirt particles; trails of ants.

Essential oils: Peppermint, Spearmint, Citronella, Orange, Cedarwood

Aphids—These colonizing pests attach to plants and feed on the nutrient-rich sap, especially the young, tender growth. They also carry harmful viruses and attract mold and other pests with their own sweet secretions.[9]

Look for: clusters of rice-sized insects which can be pink, green, black or yellow, located on the underside of tender new growth and flower buds. They prefer ornamental plants including roses.

Essential oils: Peppermint, Spearmint, Tea Tree, Eucalyptus, Hyssop, Cedarwood, Orange, Balsam Fir

Beetles—There are a variety of beetles that feed on fruits, vegetables, flowers, stems, and even roots of plants.[10]

Look for: large, irregularly-shaped holes in leaves, stems, flowers, and fruits of plants.

Essential oils: Peppermint, Thyme, Lemongrass, Cedarwood

Cabbage Loopers—These caterpillars chew ragged holes in the leaves and bore into developing heads of cabbages, broccoli, Brussels sprouts, and cauliflower.[11]

Look for: inchworm-like, pale green caterpillars; irregular holes in the leaves of plants or holes bored into heads of vegetables.

Essential oil: Rosemary

Caterpillars—Various types feed on leaves, stems, and fruit of plants.[10]

Look for: large holes chewed in leaves of plants. Some caterpillars, like the tomato hornworm, can strip all the leaves from a plant in a short amount of time. Also look for the presence of small black droppings on leaves.

Essential oils: Peppermint, Spearmint

Chiggers—Actually mites that feed on human and animal skin cells during the larval stage and on plant material in mature stages. Chiggers live in tall, grassy areas, in wooded areas, and in dense bushes or brush. They are most active on spring, summer, and fall afternoons.[12]

Look for: extremely tiny, red, round mites. They tend to bite around warm, moist areas of the body, such as folds of skin and places where clothing fits tightly. Common areas for chigger bites include: around the ankles, waist, armpits, crotch, or behind the knees. Typically, you will not notice when a chigger latches on and bites; however, within a few hours of the bite, you can feel the intense itching.[13]

Essential oils: Lavender, Lemongrass, Thyme, Sage, Cedarwood

Cockroaches—Roaches do not harm plants in your garden, but some studies show that they encourage the spread of disease.[14]

Look for: various-sized flat, oval-shaped, tan to dark brown beetles. Cockroach droppings resemble coffee grounds. The amount of droppings seen can indicate the level of infestation.

Essential oils: Eucalyptus, Peppermint, Cinnamon

Cutworms—Emerge at night and curl around plant stalks, especially those of seedlings, and chew stalks until they are cut through.[15]

Look for: caterpillars curled around the stem of plants, especially after dusk. During the day, cutworms hide in the soil near the plants upon which they feed. Adult cutworms are dark-colored moths that are active at night.

Essential oils: Thyme, Sage

Fleas—These pests do not feed on plants or other vegetation, but they are a nuisance to pets and people.

Look for: excessive itching in dogs, cats, and other pets. "Flea dirt", or droppings, near the pet's skin, as well as itchy red bites on humans and animals.[16]

Essential oils: Lavender, Lemongrass, Purification®, Cedarwood

Gnats—While gnats do not feed on plants, their larvae do eat the tender roots of plants and contribute to the spread of disease. Swarms of these tiny, flying insects can be a nuisance to the gardener as well. They are especially attracted to moist soils, so proper drainage will help to keep gnats under control.[17]

Look for: presence of large numbers of small flying insects. Affected plants may have yellowing of leaves, decreased output, and general lack of vigor. Also look for small brown scars on roots and/or root hairs being eaten off.

Essential oils: Spearmint, Patchouli, Purification®

Mice—These creatures will dig and burrow in the garden, destroying underground plantings and eating root vegetables, like carrots and potatoes, as well as newly sown seeds and flower bulbs. They also encourage the spread of many diseases, some of which are transmittable to humans and pets.[18]

Look for: small, black, rice-shaped droppings or holes in the ground, especially around the roots of plants.

Essential oil: Peppermint

Moths—While moths do not typically feed on plant material, their larvae (worms) can be quite destructive. Worms will devour leaves, flowers, and tender shoots on plants, and some even burrow into fruits and vegetables to eat the edible flesh from the inside out.

Look for: signs of worms, small clusters of eggs on the underside of leaves.

Essential oils: Lavender, Peppermint, Hyssop, Spearmint, Cedarwood

Mosquitos—These buzzing insects do not pose any harm to your garden. In fact, they provide a food source for many beneficial creatures including birds and bats. However, the nuisance they create with their itchy bite and the threat of the diseases they potentially spread is enough to make most gardeners take precautions to eliminate them. Like many other flying insects, they look for moist environments in which to lay their eggs, so good soil drainage and removal of all standing water will help to keep them under control.[19]

Look for: small larvae worms in standing water. Mosquito bites produce an itchy, raised red bump.

Essential oils: Lavender, Lemongrass, Peppermint, Purification®, Citronella

Plant Lice—These tiny insects multiply rapidly and can devastate a plant quickly. They feed mostly on leaves and stems of vegetation. Their preferred crops seem to be vegetable plants, especially tomatoes, squash, cucumbers, and carrots.[20]

Look for: groups of tiny bugs on the underside of leaves and the clear, sticky residue they leave behind.

Essential oils: Peppermint, Spearmint

Slugs & Snails—Actually mollusks, snails and slugs will feast on just about any plant. They seem to prefer young, tender transplants, leafy vegetables, and succulent plants. They are active mostly at night and during wet weather. Slugs and snails are very prolific and can lay up to 500 eggs per year.[21]

Look for: large, irregularly-shaped holes in leaves and shiny slime trails.

Essential oils for slugs: Balsam Fir, Pine, Cedarwood, Hyssop, Purification®

Essential oils for snails: Patchouli, Balsam Fir, Pine, Cedarwood

Snakes—Although snakes evoke feelings of fear for many people, they are usually a sign of a healthy garden because they prey on rodents, slugs, and other garden pests. Despite popular belief, snakes will typically avoid encounters with people, and very few of them are poisonous. If you want to deter snakes from entering certain areas, try the essential oil mixture below.[22]

Look for: shed skins of snakes or burrows in the ground. Be cautious around piles of debris, leaves, rocks, or wood, as these provide habitat for many types of snakes.

Essential oils: Mixture of equal parts Clove, Eucalyptus, Tea Tree, Lavender, and Sandalwood

Spider Mites—There are numerous kinds of spider mites that feed on plants. They prefer hot, dry conditions, so regular watering will help to discourage colonies from forming.

Look for: dense congregations of tiny mites in webs on the undersides of leaves and/or a silvering or speckled effect on leaves.[23]

Essential oils: Peppermint, Spearmint

Spiders—Many people fear spiders unnecessarily, right along with snakes. They are actually beneficial to your garden because of their voracious appetites for many garden pests. They are very effective predators, and if you learn to identify the few dangerous ones, they are not a concern. Spiders can be more of a nuisance inside the home, however.[24]

Look for: spider webs and small egg sacs on plants, buildings, and over holes in the ground.

Essential oil: Peppermint

Squash Bugs—Often referred to as "leaf bugs" because they resemble dried leaves, squash bugs will feed on many vegetable plants, with a strong preference for pumpkin and other squash plants. They suck juices from leaves, causing them to dry up and turn black.

Look for: leaf-shaped and colored bugs; shriveled, blackened leaves, reduced output of a plant.[25]

Essential oils: Peppermint

Ticks—These parasites tend to live in grassy or wooded areas. They do not pose a threat to garden plants, but they do feed on the blood of humans and pets, and they spread dangerous diseases including Lyme disease and Rocky Mountain spotted fever. No beneficial attributes of ticks have been found.[26]

Look for: small, round brown/black bugs attached to people or pets, especially in warm, moist areas, such as the armpits, groin, or scalp, and around face and ears of pets.

Essential oils: Lavender, Lemongrass, Purification®, Sage, Thyme, Citronella

Weevils—There are two types of these beetles: vine weevils and root weevils. Vine weevils feed predominantly on vines and leaves of plants.[27] While adult root weevils will feed on the tops of plants, the real damage is caused by the immature larvae, which feed on roots and root vegetables, often resulting in death of the plant.[28]

Look for: white grubs in the soil and/or long-legged beetle-like insects with a long proboscis (snout). In addition to root damage, leaves of affected plants may be irregularly shaped and wilted.

Essential oils: Patchouli, Cedarwood

Whiteflies—These tiny insects suck plant juices from the leaves and stems of almost any plant. They secrete a sticky, sweet substance that can encourage some types of fungus to grow.[29]

Look for: small, triangularly-shaped white insects with transparent wings that tend to congregate on the undersides of leaves near the veins. Eggs and tiny oval-shaped larvae may also be seen on the undersides of leaves. Ants are attracted to their sweet, sticky secretions, so the presence of ants can also alert to a whitefly infestation. Affected plants will become weak with wilted or yellowed leaves and stunted growth.[30]

Essential oils: Peppermint, Tea Tree

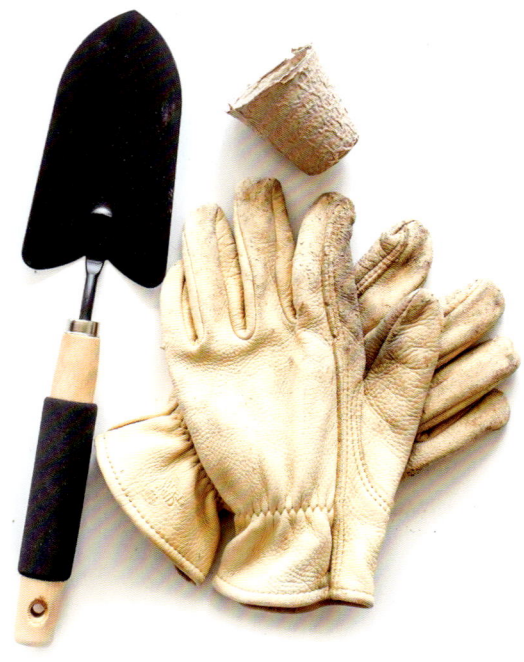

QUICK-REFERENCE CHART OF GARDEN PESTS & ESSENTIAL OIL REMEDIES[31]

Pest	Essential Oils
Ants	Peppermint, Spearmint, Citronella, Orange, Cedarwood
Aphids	Peppermint, Spearmint, Tea Tree, Eucalyptus, Hyssop, Cedarwood, Orange, Balsam Fir
Beetles	Peppermint, Thyme, Lemongrass, Cedarwood
Cabbage Loopers	Rosemary
Caterpillars	Peppermint, Spearmint
Chiggers	Lavender, Lemongrass, Thyme, Sage, Cedarwood
Cockroaches	Eucalyptus, Peppermint, Cinnamon
Cutworms	Thyme, Sage
Fleas	Lavender, Lemongrass, Purification®, Cedarwood
Flies	Lavender, Peppermint, Purification®, Thieves®, Basil, Clove, Eucalyptus Globulus, Rosemary, Citronella
Gnats	Spearmint, Patchouli, Purification®
Mice	Peppermint
Moths	Lavender, Peppermint, Hyssop, Spearmint, Cedarwood
Mosquitoes	Lavender, Lemongrass, Peppermint, Purification®, Citronella
Plant Lice	Peppermint, Spearmint
Slugs	Balsam Fir, Pine, Cedarwood, Hyssop, Purification®
Snails	Patchouli, Balsam Fir, Pine, Cedarwood
Snakes	Mixture of Clove, Eucalyptus, Tea Tree, Lavender, and Sandalwood
Spider Mites	Peppermint, Spearmint
Spiders	Peppermint
Squash Bugs	Peppermint
Ticks	Lavender, Lemongrass, Purification®, Sage, Thyme, Citronella
Weevils	Patchouli, Cedarwood
White Flies	Peppermint, Tea Tree

Broad-Spectrum Garden Pest Control Spray
Use this all-purpose spray to prevent and control a variety of common garden intruders.

10 drops Peppermint essential oil
10 drops Thyme essential oil
10 drops Clove essential oil
Gallon of water

Combine and spray liberally on and around plants.

Fire Ant Spray
16 drops Peppermint essential oil
5 drops Cinnamon essential oil
10 drops Orange essential oil
5 drops Wintergreen essential oil
Pint of water

Combine and spray directly on anthills or infested areas.

Deer and Rabbit Repellent
20 drops Clove essential oil
1 cup sour cream or buttermilk
2 raw eggs—beaten
1 tsp cooking oil
1 tsp. dish soap or castile soap
One cup of water

Combine ingredients in a mixer or blender. Add to a one-gallon sprayer and top off with water. Spray plants or around the garden area you want to protect. Apply every two weeks or after a heavy rain.

Squirrel and Chipmunk Repellent
Add Peppermint Oil to cotton balls and place around the garden. Replace every 3 weeks.

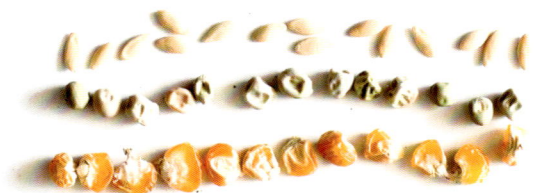

Fighting Common Diseases in the Garden with Essential Oils

Essential oils are invaluable when it comes to dealing with garden diseases. Many essential oils have antibacterial, antifungal, and antiseptic properties.

FUNGUS

Garden fungus, including mold and mildew, is responsible for about 85% of all plant diseases. Because fungus spores are resistant to both heat and cold, a fungal infection can be difficult to treat, but there are many essential oil remedies that create an environment that is unfavorable to fungi. Because fungi prefer warm, moist conditions, maintaining good drainage and not over-watering can help to prevent fungal outbreaks.

Early Blight usually affects vegetables and fruit trees. Plants under stress, due to extreme weather or improper nutrition, or those with a heavy load of fruit are most susceptible. Symptoms include large brown and black spots on leaves; symptoms usually appear on lower leaves first.[32]

Late Blight usually affects tomatoes, peppers and potatoes. Symptoms include water-soaked spots on top of leaves with white, fuzzy growth on the underside. Late blight also appears on lower leaves of the plant first.[33]

Powdery Mildew is a powdery, white growth that grows on the surface of leaves. The fungus robs the plant of necessary nutrients, which causes loss of leaves, reduced yield of produce, and even death of the plant.[34]

Club Root affects vegetables in the cabbage family. The infected plants will wilt, and older leaves will turn yellow and drop. It also distorts the roots and stunts the growth of the plant. This fungus favors warm, wet soil and left untreated, can live in the soil for up to ten years.[35]

Gray Mold spreads rapidly in gardens, especially during damp, cool weather. Symptoms include soft, gray, mushy spots on leaves, stems, flowers and on produce. Fuzzy, gray fungus spores will eventually cover spots, resulting in shriveling and rotting of fruit and plants.[36]

Tomato Blight Recipe

3 drops Purification® essential oil
1 drop Oregano essential oil
Pint of water

Combine oils and water and spray affected plant(s).

Club Root Remedy

Lemon, Oregano and/or Tea Tree essential oil
Quart of water

Add 8-10 drops of essential oil to one quart of water. Spray liberally around affected plant(s).

Gray Mold Remedy

1 capful of Thieves® Cleaner
Quart of water

Remove affected leaves and/or fruit from plants. Combine Thieves® cleaner with water and spray liberally over entire plant and surrounding soil.

General Fungi Treatment

Essential oils: Tea Tree (first choice), Citronella, Rosemary, Peppermint or Thieves®
1 quart of water
1 Tbsp. baking soda
1 drop mild dishwashing liquid or castile soap

Combine 8-10 drops of essential oil(s), baking soda, and dishwashing liquid. Shake thoroughly before applying to affected plant(s). Apply once or twice a week as needed.

BACTERIA

Most bacterial diseases are spread by garden pests, especially sap-sucking insects, because they typically infect plants through natural openings or wounds. Bacteria multiply within the infected plants and can live in the soil and plant debris around plants as well. Again, proper drainage, along with keeping your garden clean, will help to prevent serious bacterial infections.[37]

Bacterial Wilts will cause large, light green spots on leaves that later turn yellow and can cause the leaves to fall off. Spots will often produce yellow ooze or appear as dead spots with yellow halos around them. This bacterium is commonly found in the gut of cucumber beetles.[38]

Bacterial Wilt Treatment

8-10 drops of Purification®, Rosemary, Oregano, Thyme or Tea Tree essential oil (or a combination)
Quart of water

First remove any affected leaves or stems. Add 8-10 drops of essential oils to one quart of water, and spray liberally over affected plant(s).

Natural Weed Control with Essential Oils

Many weeds are naturally discouraged by a garden that is healthy and thriving, but the occasional weed is inevitable with any type of garden. A layer of mulch over the soil surface can prevent many weeds from taking root. The simplest method of removing weeds is pulling them out by hand as they appear in the garden. Below is a recipe you can use to combat stubborn weeds or a more widespread problem.

BASIC WEED KILLER

Essential oils: Cinnamon Bark, Palo Santo, Basil, Pine, or Plectranthus Oregano
20 oz. white vinegar
1 drop castile soap

According to Gary Young, "Commercial sprays are not used on Young Living essential oil crops period, irrespective of what other people out there may say." Instead, farm workers painstakingly hand-pull and use essential oil blends to spray individual weeds by hand.[39]

Combine 8-10 drops of selected essential oil, vinegar, and soap. Shake thoroughly before applying to weed(s). Use caution to avoid spraying the soil or surrounding plants.

Companion Gardening with Essential Oils

Companion planting with vegetables, herbs, and flowers is based on the idea that certain crops planted together have a beneficial partnership. Companion plants assist the growth of one another by attracting beneficial insects, repelling pests, providing nutrients, and conserving space. Thus, companion planting can reduce the time and effort involved in pest control and improves the health and yield of the plants.

ESSENTIAL OILS AS COMPANIONS

As described in the "What are Essential Oils" section (p. 5), plants have very complex chemical processes that combat pests, disease, and natural elements. They have constituents that work as insecticides, fungicides, antivirals, and antibiotics, in addition to other defense substances.[38] Because these substances are all contained in the essential oil of the plants, applying the oils directly to plants in the garden proves to be a very efficient and low-maintenance solution. Thus, essential oils and plants become great companions in gardening.

SOIL ENHANCER

Amend soil with Lavender essential oil to improve the growing conditions of plants. Sprinkle a few drops on the soil around plants or mix into compost before spreading in the garden. Alternatively, you can add 2-3 drops to the watering can for regular watering.

BASIC COMPANION SOLUTION

6-8 drops of essential oils (select from chart on the next page)
2 gallons of water

Combine oils and water and apply solution liberally to plants and the surrounding soil. Be careful not to apply to foliage during the heat of the day. For best results, apply the companion mixture 1-2 times weekly.

ESSENTIAL OILS AND THE PLANTS THEY BENEFIT[40]

Plant	Essential Oil(s)
Apples	Lavender, Marjoram, Melissa
Asparagus	Basil
Beans	Rosemary, Basil
Beets	Dill, Rosemary, Geranium, Thyme
Broccoli	Basil, Thyme, Rosemary, Sage, Dill
Cabbage	Peppermint, Coriander, Rosemary, Chamomile, Thyme, Sage, Hyssop
Carrots	Peppermint, Thyme, Sage, Rosemary
Cauliflower	Thyme, Sage
Cucumbers	Chamomile, Oregano, Sage
Eggplants	Peppermint, Spearmint, Thyme
Grapes	Lavender, Hyssop
Leeks	Celery, Hyssop
Lettuce	Chamomile, Cilantro, Thyme, Carrot
Melons	Oregano
Okra	Basil
Onion	Chamomile
Peas	Geranium, Peppermint, Spearmint, Carrot
Peppers	Marjoram, Geranium, Basil
Potatoes	Basil, Sage
Petunias	Basil
Pumpkins	Oregano
Squash	Peppermint, Oregano, Dill
Roses	Basil, Hyssop, Thyme
Strawberries	Thyme
Sweet Potatoes	Dill, Thyme, Oregano
Tomatoes	Basil, Peppermint

Attracting Natural Pollinators with Essential Oils

Just as you can use essential oils to repel pests in the garden, they can also be used attract natural pollinators. Choose one or more essential oils from the lists below and use the cotton ball, hanging cloth strips, or string method of application. (See p. 12.)

BEES
Orange, Coriander, Lemongrass, Lavender, Hyssop, Marjoram, Helichrysum, Basil, Sage, Roman Chamomile, Rosemary, Dill

BUTTERFLIES
Lavender, Mint, Fennel, Sage, Helichrysum

OTHER BENEFICIAL INSECTS (such as ladybugs, hoverflies, lacewings, parasitic wasps)
Coriander, Dill, Fennel, Roman Chamomile

POLLINATOR'S FAVORITE BLEND RECIPE
12 drops Lavender essential oil
8 drops Rosemary essential oil
5 drops Orange essential oil

Combine oils and add to cotton balls, string or cloth strips, and scatter in the garden around plants.

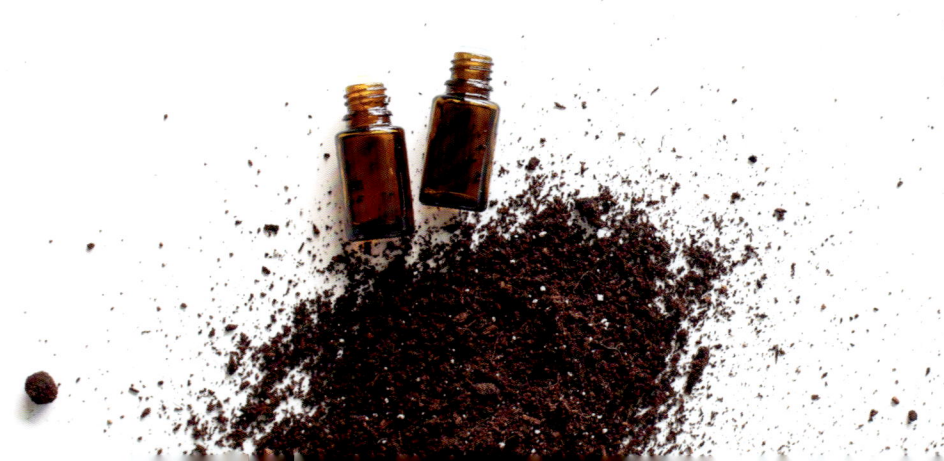

Essential Oils for the Gardener

GARDENING AS THERAPY

Nature has long been known for its relaxing qualities, as a place for humans to find tranquility and healing. Gardening, in particular, is associated with mental clarity and feelings of reward, and it has many physical benefits as well. Fruit and vegetable gardening can be particularly gratifying and provide an excellent source of healthy, fresh produce. In addition to these benefits, gardening is great exercise for the body as well as the mind.[41]

According to the Centers for Disease Control and Prevention (CDC), 2-1/2 hours of moderate-intensity level activity can reduce the risk of obesity, high blood pressure, type 2 diabetes, osteoporosis, heart disease, stroke, depression, colon cancer, and premature death. The CDC considers gardening a moderate-intensity level activity.[41]

Gardening has also emerged in recent years as a scientifically proven stress reliever. Stress wreaks havoc on the body and can cause irritability, headaches, stomachaches, heart attacks, and other health issues.[41]

If you are a gardener, you know how gardening can benefit both the body and the soul. However, gardening can come with some potential hazards if you're not careful. There are risks of accidental cuts and scrapes, sunburn, overexertion, skin irritations, insect bites, respiratory issues and other discomforts. Thankfully, there are some simple precautions you can take to avoid most gardening hazards, and the same essential oils that help your garden bloom can help you stay healthy as well.

PREVENTING GARDENING MISHAPS

- Stretch before you work to prepare your muscles, prevent injury, and limit soreness.
- Wear gloves, a hat, and long sleeved shirt and apply sunscreen to protect against the elements of sun, water, and other hazards.
- When using machinery, wear safety glasses and earplugs to protect your eyes and ears. If you are not familiar with the use of a gardening device, seek proper training, or leave it to the experts.
- Protect your knees and back! Lift with proper techniques and consider wearing kneepads for kneeling in your garden.

- Know your limitations. Take frequent breaks and remember to stay hydrated while working. Rotate your tasks and change positions frequently to give muscles time to recuperate.
- Consider creating a gardening first aid kit to have handy, complete with basic implements, bandages and remedies from this booklet.
- Be sure to wash your hands thoroughly after gardening, especially before eating.
- Keep the garden tidy to avoid trips and falls. Remember to put away all garden tools, especially where curious children might investigate.

DID YOU KNOW ESSENTIAL OILS...
- Enhance your mood
- Support overall health and wellness
- Promote relaxation and sleep
- Heal skin irritations
- Relieve inflammation
- And much more!

HOW TO USE ESSENTIAL OILS
The three standard methods of application are topically, aromatically, and internally.

Topically
Essential oils are safe and beneficial to apply directly on the skin. Oils can be applied neat (without a carrier oil) or diluted, based on personal preference and skin sensitivity.

Aromatically
Breathing in the aroma of essential oils can deliver great health benefits. A cold-air diffuser is a great way to enjoy the aroma of oils, or simply place a few drops in your hands, cup your hands around your nose, and inhale.

Internally
Young Living's Vitality™ essential oils are labeled for culinary and dietary use. These oils can be added to water or other beverages, used in recipes, or swallowed in capsules.

Common Gardeners' Ailments

THINGS THAT BITE!

Bee, Wasp, and Hornet Stings

These stings can be painful and annoying. If the stinger remains in the skin, numb the affected area with one drop of Clove essential oil before removing. In the case of an allergic reaction to a sting, seek medical attention immediately.

Essential oil recommendations: Lavender, Peppermint, Purification®, Chamomile, Vetiver

Application: Combine 2 drops of chosen essential oil with 1 tsp. baking soda to form a paste. Apply to sting and allow to dry. This can be repeated every 20 minutes until discomfort is relieved.

Chigger and Tick Bites

It is important that ticks and chiggers be removed before treating the bite. Mix one drop each of Thyme and Oregano essential oils and apply over the bite area. The high phenol content of the oils will cause the tick or chigger to release.

Essential oil recommendations: Peppermint, Lavender, Rosemary, Myrrh, Frankincense, Idaho Balsam Fir, Purification®, Melrose™, Thieves®

Application: Apply 1-3 drops of selected essential oils, neat or diluted, to affected area 1-3 times daily.

Other Minor Bites & Stings

Essential oil recommendations: Lavender, Purification®, Peppermint, Melrose™, Thieves®, Tea Tree, Rosemary, Frankincense

Application: Apply a dab of selected essential oil to affected area for immediate relief.

Snake Bites

If you are bitten by a venomous snake, seek medical attention immediately. Even a non-venomous snakebite can be painful and susceptible to infection.

Essential oil recommendations: Thieves®, Lavender, Oregano, Clove, Idaho Balsam Fir, Copaiba, Sacred Frankincense™, Tea Tree, Purification®, PanAway®

Application: Thieves® or Oregano oil can be applied directly to a recent bite to prevent infection. Other oils may bring relief from pain and irritation of affected area.

Spider Bites

If you suspect you have been bitten by a black widow or brown recluse spider, seek medical attention immediately.

Essential oil recommendations: Lavender, Eucalyptus, Tea Tree, Peppermint, Myrrh, Frankincense, Rosemary, Thieves®, PanAway®

Application: Apply selected essential oil(s) to the bite to relieve pain, reduce inflammation, and prevent infection. If serious infection develops, or nausea, muscle cramps, vomiting, joint pain, or severe abdominal pain occurs, seek medical attention.

OUCH! INEVITABLE GARDENING ACCIDENTS

Bruising

Bruising is caused by a break in capillary walls.

Essential oil recommendations: Helichrysum, Geranium, Lavender, Lemongrass, Deep Relief™ Roll-On, PanAway®

Application: Apply 1-4 drops of selected essential oil(s) to affected area 2-3 times daily.

Burns and Blisters

Caused by sunlight, chemicals, electricity, heat and friction, burns, and blisters are a common complaint of most active gardeners.

Essential oil recommendations: Lavender, Helichrysum, Roman Chamomile, Idaho Balsam Fir, Tea Tree, LavaDerm™ Cooling Mist

Application: Apply 1-5 drops selected essential oil(s) to affected area 2-3 times daily. If the area is very sensitive or if you need to cover a large area, you can dilute essential oils with a carrier oil, such as coconut, almond, olive oil, or Young Living's V-6™ blend. LavaDerm™ Cooling Mist is very soothing and can be used liberally to manage discomfort.

Cuts and Scrapes

Essential oil recommendations: Lavender, Helichrysum, Frankincense, Myrrh, Rosemary, Thieves® Spray, LavaDerm™ Cooling Mist

Application: Apply 1-4 drops of selected essential oil(s), neat or diluted, to affected area 1-3 times daily. Thieves® Spray can be used to disinfect the area, and LavaDerm™ Cooling Mist is very soothing.

Poison Oak/Poison Ivy/Poison Sumac

These plants contain oil called urushiol, which triggers an allergic reaction when it comes into contact the skin. Accidentally touching one of these plants can result in an itchy, painful rash within hours or even several days after exposure, and it usually develops into oozing blisters. The oil from these plants can be transmitted via garden tools, shoes, and even pets. If you encounter a poisonous plant, scrub the affected area immediately with hot water and soap to avoid a serious reaction and the chance of spreading the oil.

Essential oil recommendations: Myrrh, Eucalyptus, Rose, Tee Tree, Cypress, Peppermint, Purification®, Roman Chamomile, Lavender, Rose Ointment™, Thieves® Spray, LavaDerm™ Cooling Mist, ClaraDerm™ Spray

Application: Apply selected essential oil(s) to affected areas. Oils may be also added to Young Living's Rose Ointment™ or another carrier oil if desired. Thieves® Spray can be used to cleanse the area and remove urushiol oil from the plant. LavaDerm™ Cooling Mist and ClaraDerm™ Spray may relieve pain and itching.

Poison Ivy Relief

4 tsp. water
2 tsp. Himalayan pink salt
3 tsp. apple cider vinegar
2 drops Roman Chamomile essential oil
6 drops Tea Tree essential oil
5 drops Lavender essential oil
4 drops Peppermint essential oil

Mix all ingredients thoroughly in a small glass jar. Apply liberally to poison ivy, oak, or sumac rash 3-4 times daily while symptoms persist.

General Itching

Itching can be due to dry skin, insect bites, allergies or overexposure to chemicals or sunlight.

Essential oil recommendations: Lavender, German Chamomile, Patchouli, Melrose™, Purification®, Palmarosa

Application: Apply 1-3 drops of chosen essential oil(s), neat or diluted, to affected area. For widespread itching, add 2 cups Epsom salt and a few drops of essential oil to a warm bath.

IT GOES WITH THE TERRITORY

Chapped, Cracked, or Dry Skin

Dry, chapped skin results from the loss of the protective lipid layer on the skin surface. In severe cases, skin may also crack and become more susceptible to infection.

Essential oil recommendations: Carrot Seed, Frankincense, Rose, Cedarwood, Patchouli, Geranium, Lavender, Myrrh, Sandalwood

Healing Body Butter

Use this recipe to create a creamy, soothing lotion for cracked, chapped hands and feet.

1/2 cup organic coconut oil
1/2 cup organic, unrefined shea butter
10 drops Melrose™ essential oil
10 drops Lavender essential oil

Whip coconut oil and shea butter until creamy. Add essential oils and whip again to thoroughly combine. Store in a glass jar away from direct light.

Hay Fever/Allergies

Airborne allergens (pollen, animal hair, feathers, dust mites, etc.) can cause the release of histamines and uncomfortable inflammation of nasal passages and sinus area.

Essential oil recommendations: R.C.™, Raven™, Lavender, Eucalyptus Blue, Eucalyptus Radiata, Peppermint, Frankincense, Lemon

Application: Diffuse, inhale, or topically apply chosen essential oil(s) during times of discomfort.

Hay Fever Blend:

3 drops Lemon Vitality™
3 drops Lavender Vitality™
3 drops Peppermint Vitality™

Combine oils in a vegetable capsule and swallow. Alternatively, diffuse or rub oils in hands and inhale.

Muscle Soreness—A day of strenuous activity in the garden can create muscle soreness.

Essential oil recommendations: PanAway®, Deep Rel ef™ Roll-on, Aroma Siez™, Cool Azul™ Pain Relief Cream, Rosemary, Peppermint, Idaho Balsam Fir, Copaiba

Application: Apply 1-6 drops of selected essential oil(s) to affected area as needed. A carrier oil can also be added to create a pain-relieving massage oil. A warm bath with 2-3 cups of Epsom salt and 3-6 drops of essential oils is very soothing after a long day of working in the garden.

Sore Muscle Blend

5 drops Idaho Balsam Fir essential oil
5 drops Copaiba essential oil
5 drops Frankincense essential oil

Combine oils in a vegetable capsule and swallow. May be repeated up to 3 times daily. Alternatively, combine oils in 2 oz. of carrier oil, such as coconut, almond, olive oil, or Young Living's V-6™ blend, and massage into sore muscles.

RECIPES

Gardener's Hand Scrub

This moisturizing scrub will leave hands smooth and clean. The avocado oil conditions hands, so there is no need to moisturize afterwards.

1 oz. (30ml) avocado oil
1 oz. (28g) pink Himalayan salt, or any medium-grain salt
7 drops Rosemary essential oil
10 drops Basil essential oil

In a 2-ounce jar, combine salt and avocado oil. Add essential oils and stir gently. Use a small amount to scrub and exfoliate hands. Rinse and dry.

Gardener's Hand Cream

4 oz. organic, unrefined shea butter
3 Tbsp. organic, extra-virgin olive oil or sunflower oil
2 tsp. cornstarch or arrowroot powder
20 drops essential oils—Suggestions: Lavender, Peppermint, Orange, or Lemongrass

Using an electric mixer, whip shea butter until light and fluffy. Add olive oil and cornstarch, and whip again until thoroughly combined. Scrape down the sides of your bowl and add 20 drops of essential oil. Whip a final time until fluffy. Store in two 4 oz. jars in a cool, dark location.

Bath Salts

Use this recipe to soak away tiredness, decrease stress, improve mental clarity, relieve muscle soreness, help with sinus congestion, and support body detoxification.

2 cups Epsom salt
1/2 cup baking soda
10-15 drops of essential oils (choose from below)

Mix together and add to warm bath water.

Essential Oil Bath Blends:
Just Relax—Lavender, Bergamot, Stress Away™
Happy Muscles—Eucalyptus, Rosemary, PanAway®
Take a Deep Breath—Eucalyptus, Peppermint, R.C.™
Wake up and Smell the Roses—Rosemary, Citrus Fresh™, Peppermint

Foot Soak

Treat your tired, worn out feet to this luxurious, relaxing foot soak.

1/4 cup Epsom salt
2 drops Lime essential oil
2 drops Peppermint essential oil

Fill a small tub with enough warm water to cover your feet up to the ankles. Add Epsom salt and oils. Soak feet for 30-60 minutes. Other essential oils may be substituted as desired.

OTHER HELPFUL TIPS:

Insect Repellent
Purification® or Citronella oil can be applied topically to keep stinging and biting pests away. Also try Young Living's plant-based Insect Repellent.

Cool-off
A couple drops of Peppermint oil applied to the back of the neck brings cooling relief. You can also make a refreshing spray:

> Combine 10 drops Peppermint essential oil with 4 oz. water in a spray bottle. Use liberally to keep cool, avoiding the eyes.

Cleaning Fresh Produce
Lemon oil offers a simple way to clean produce without adding unnecessary chemicals found in soaps and other cleaners. The lemon oil will help to extend the life of your fruits and vegetables by inhibiting mold and bacteria. Simply fill a basin or bowl with water and add a drop or two of lemon oil. Soak your bounty for 2-3 minutes, drain anc air dry. Also try Young Living Thieves® Fruit and Veggie Wash or Spray.

Cleaning Garden Tools
Tea Tree oil is very effective for cleaning garden tools and around the greenhouse because it prevents fungus and bacteria contamination.

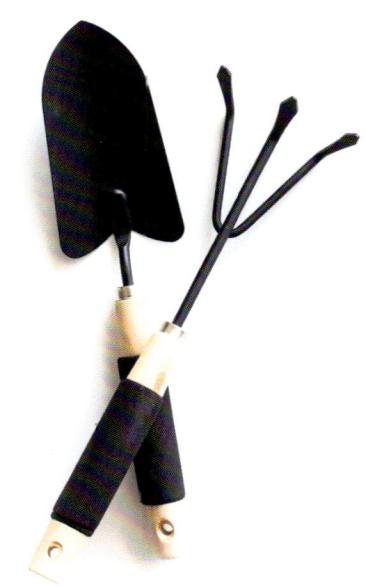

> Use a mixture of 10 drops of oil to 32 ounces of water to clean all kinds of surfaces, pots, garden tools, and other implements.

Prolong the Life of Cut Flowers
Try adding a drop of Purification® to the water in your vase to lengthen the life of cut flowers.

References

1. Mercola, Joseph. (2015, June 6). "Documentary Reveals How Prolific Chemicals are in Our Daily Lives". Retrieved from: https://articles.mercola.com/sites/articles/archive/2015/06/06/chemical-exposure.aspx.

2. Vinje, E. (2013). "Lawn and Garden Chemicals" Retrieved from: https://www.planetnatural.com/garden-chemicals/.

3. "Radioactive Material from Fertilizer Production". Retrieved from: https://www3.epa.gov/radtown/fertilizer-production.html.

4. Barrett, Abbie. (2008, May). "A Beginner's Guide to Organic Gardening". Retrieved from: http://www.wholeliving.com/134279/beginners-guide-organic-gardening.

5. *Planet Natural.* Retrieved from: https://www.planetnatural.com/composting-101/.

6. Young, Gary D. (2013, October 31). "Composting and Worm Castings". Retrieved from: https://www.dgaryyoung.com/blog/2013/composting-and-worm-castings/.

7. Young, Gary D. (2013, November 7). "Worm Housed Enrich Farm Soil". Retrieved from: https://www.dgaryyoung.com/blog/2013/worm-houses-enrich-farm-soil/.

8. *VeggieGardener.com.* (2009, June 18). "Are Ants in the Vegetable Garden a Bad Thing?" Retrieved from: http://www.veggiegardener.com/are-ants-in-the-vegetable-garden-a-bad-thing/.

9. National Gardening Association Editors. "Pest Control Library: Aphids". Retrieved from: https://garden.org/learn/articles/view/1586/.

10. National Gardening Association Editors. "Pest Control Library". Retrieved from: https://garden.org/learn/library/pests/

11. National Gardening Association Editors. "Pest Control Library: Cabbage Loopers". Retrieved from: https://garden.org/learn/articles/view/1592/.

12. PestProducts.com "Chiggers". Retrieved from: http://www.pestproducts.com/chiggers.htm.

13. Pietrangelo, Ann. (2016, December 9). "Chiggers: Little Bugs with a Big Bite". Retrieved from: https://www.healthline.com/health/chigger-bites#symptoms.

14. Littlefield, Susan. "Take Two Cockroaches and Call Me in the Morning". Retrieved from: https://garden.org/learn/articles/view/3368/.

15. *National Gardening Association Editors.* "Pest Control Library: Cutworm". Retrieved from: https://garden.org/learn/articles/view/1604/.

16. WebMD Veterinary Reference from ASPCA Virtual Pet Behaviorist (2015-2018). "Fleas on Dogs: What to Look For". Retrieved from: https://pets.webmd.com/dogs/guide/fleas-dogs-what-look-for#1.

17. Blackstone, Victoria Lee. "Are Tiny Gnats From Soil Harmful to Plants?" Retrieved from: http://homeguides.sfgate.com/tiny-gnats-soil-harmful-plants-70291.html.

18. National Pest Management Association. (2014, November 24). "Health Hazards Posed by Rodents". Retrieved from: https://www.pestworld.org/news-hub/pest-health-hub/health-hazards-posed-by-rodents/.

19. Schmidt, Genevieve. (2014, June 8). "Don't Bug Me! How to Get Rid of Mosquitos in the Garden". Retrieved from: http://northcoastgardening.com/2014/06/mosquito-repelling-garden/.

20. Balarini, Elizabeth. (2017, September 21). "Vegetable Gardens and Plant Lice". Retrieved from: https://www.gardenguides.com/90017-vegetable-gardens-plant-lice.html.

21. *National Gardening Association Editors.* "Pest Control Library: Slugs and Snails". Retrieved from: https://garden.org/learn/articles/view/1748/.

22. *National Gardening Association Editors.* "Pest Control Library: Snakes". Retrieved from: https://garden.org/learn/articles/view/1800/.

23. *National Gardening Association Editors.* "Pest Control Library: Spider Mites". Retrieved from: https://garden.org/learn/articles/view/1633/.

24. Vinje, E. "Charlotte's Web in Your Garden". Retrieved from: https://www.planetnatural.com/garden-spiders/.

25. *National Gardening Association Editors.* "Pest Control Library: Squash Bugs". Retrieved from: https://garden.org/learn/articles/view/1634/.

26. Burke, Darla. (2015, November 12). "Ticks and the Diseases They Carry". Retrieved from: https://www.healthline.com/health/tick-infestations.

27. *Royal Horticultural Society.* (2014) "Vine Weevil". Retrieved from: https://www.rhs.org.uk/advice/profile?PID=234.

28. *Gardening Know How.* "Identifying and Controlling Root Weevil". Retrieved from: https://www.gardeningknowhow.com/plant-problems/pests/insects/controlling-root-weevil.htm.

29. *National Gardening Association Editors.* "Pest Control Library: Whiteflies". Retrieved from: https://garden.org/learn/articles/view/1641/.

30. *E³Aromatherapy Solutions.* "Essential Oils for the Garden and Gardener". Retrieved from: https://essentialthree.com/essential-oils-for-the-garden-gardener/.

31. *The Old Farmer's Almanac.* (2014) Retrieved from: https://www.almanac.com/pest/whiteflies.

32. *National Gardening Association Editors.* "Pest Control Library: Early Blight". Retrieved from: https://garden.org/learn/articles/view/1783/.

33. *National Gardening Association Editors.* "Pest Control Library: Late Blight". Retrieved from: https://garden.org/learn/articles/view/1784/.

34. *National Gardening Association Editors.* "Pest Control Library: Powdery Mildew". Retrieved from: https://garden.org/learn/articles/view/1789/.

35. *National Gardening Association Editors.* "Pest Control Library: Club Root". Retrieved from: https://garden.org/learn/articles/view/1779/.

36. *Planet Natural.* "Gray Mold". Retrieved from: https://www.planetnatural.com/pest-problem-solver/plant-disease/gray-mold/.

37. Russell, Kate. (2017, November 1). "Garden Word of the Day: Bacterial Disease". Retrieved from: https://www.thedailygarden.us/garden-word-of-the-day/bacterial-disease.

38. *National Gardening Association Editors.* "Pest Control Library: Bacterial Wilt". Retrieved from: https://garden.org/learn/articles/view/1775/.

39. Young, Gary D. (2013, November 14). "Developing Organic Weed and Pest Control". Retrieved from: https://www.dgaryyoung.com/blog/2013/developing-organic-weed-and-pest-control/.

40. Oijala, Leena. (2013, March 31). "Planning a Garden: The Benefits of Companion Planting". Retrieved from: http://www.organicauthority.com/organic-gardening/planning-a-garden-companion-planting.html.

41. Darnton, Julia. (2014, May 19). "What are the Physical and Mental Benefits of Gardening?". Retrieved from: http://msue.anr.msu.edu/news/what_are_the_physical_and_mental_benefits_of_gardening.

OTHER SOURCES

Greener Ideal. (2014, August 28). "8 Simple Steps to Start Your Own Organic Garden". Retrieved from: https://greenerideal.com/guides/1229-start-an-organic-garden

Koul, Opender, Walia, Suresh, Dhaliwal, G. S. (2008, March 1). "Essential Oils as Green Pesticides: Potential and Constraints". Retrieved from: http://projects.nri.org/adappt/docs/63-84.pdf.

Mindi. (2010). "How to Fight Common Vegetable Garden Diseases Naturally Using Essential Oils". Retrieved from: http://momsneedtoknow.com/about/.

Ritz, Jackie. (2015, August 10). "Essential Oils for Your Garden". Retrieved from: https://thepaleomama.com/2015/08/10/essential-oils-for-your-garden/.

Sideman, Eric and English, Jean. (2009, April). "Basics of Organic Vegetable Gardening". Retrieved from: http://mofga.org/Portals/2/Fact%20Sheets/TB%201%20Organic%20Gardening%20Basics.pdf.